Keto Diet for Vegetarians

The Best Keto Diet for Vegetarians to Burn Fat and Lose 20 Pounds in 15 Days with Delicious Recipes.

Sebi Alan Guntry

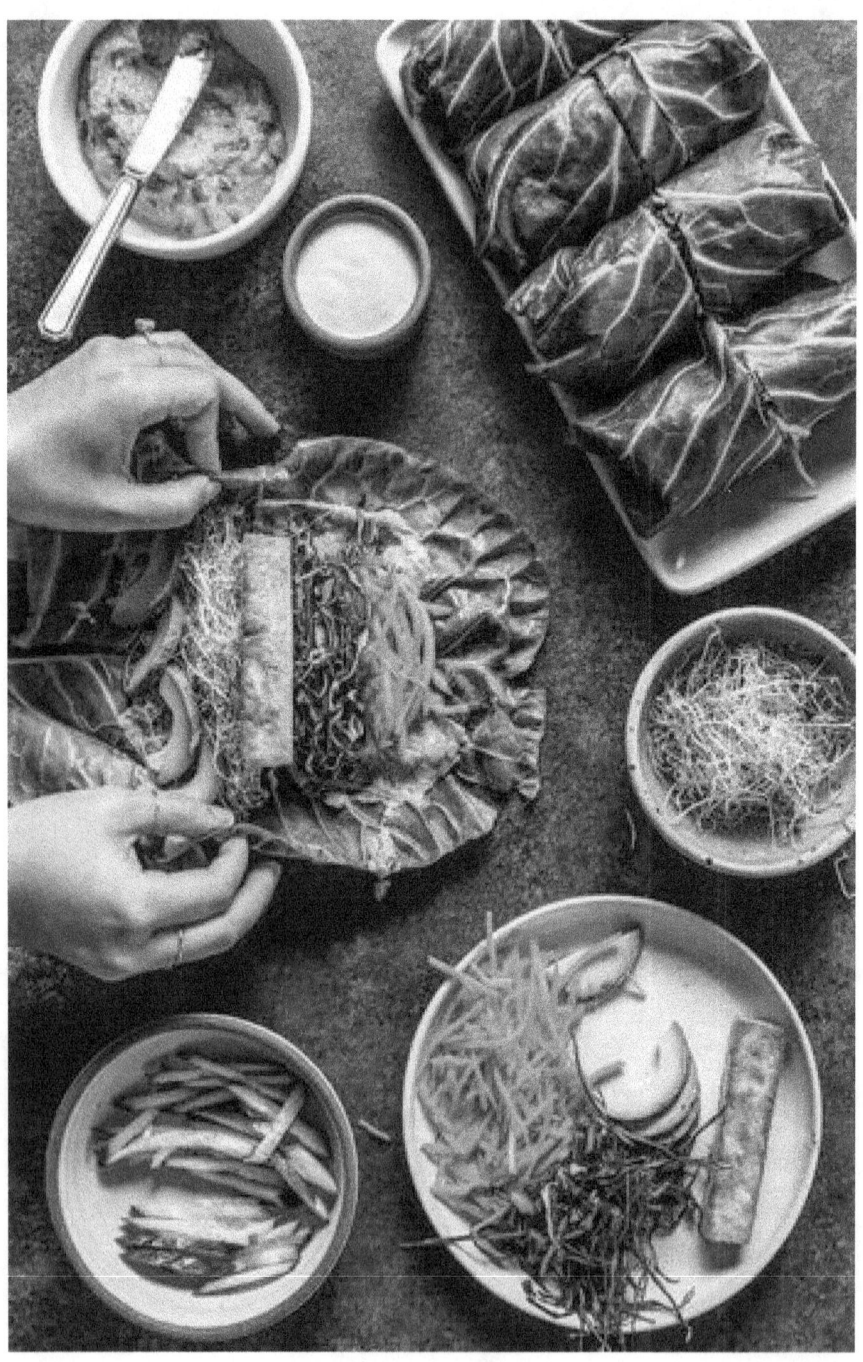

Tables of contains

INTRODUCTION 7

BREAKFAST 12
- Pumpkin pancakes 13
- Quinoa Applesauce Muffins 16
- Green breakfast smoothie 19
- Blueberry Lemonade Smoothie 21
- Berry Protein Smoothie 23
- Almond Plum Oats Overnight 25
- Avocado Miso Chickpeas Toast 28
- Banana Malt Bread 30
- Banana Vegan Bread 33
- Berry Compote Pancakes 36
- Buckwheat Crepes 39
- Chickpeas Spread Sourdough Toast 41
- Chickpeas with Harissa 43

LUNCH 45
- Whipped Potatoes 46
- Quinoa Avocado Salad 49
- Roasted Sweet Potatoes 52
- Cauliflower Salad 54
- Garlic Mashed Potatoes & Turnips 56
- Cashew Siam Salad 58
- Avocado and Cauliflower Hummus 61
- Raw Zoodles with Avocado 'N Nuts 64
- Cauliflower Sushi 66
- Spinach and Mashed Tofu Salad 69
- Cucumber Edamame Salad 72
- Artichoke White Bean Sandwich Spread 75

DINNER 78
- Curried Tofu with Buttery Cabbage 79
- Smoked Tempeh with Broccoli Fritters 81
- Cheesy Potato Casserole 85
- Spicy Cheesy Tofu Balls 90
- Greek-style Gigante Beans 92
- Brown Rice & Red Beans & Coconut Milk 94
- Black-Eyed Peas with Herns 96
- Cream of Mushroom Soup 98
- Cauliflower and Horseradish Soup 101

Curry Lentil Soup 103
Chickpea Noodle Soup 105

© Copyright 2021 by Sebi Alan Guntry - All rights reserved.

The following Book is reproduced below with the goal of providing information that is as accurate and reliable as possible. Regardless, purchasing this Book can be seen as consent to the fact that both the publisher and the author of this book are in no way experts on the topics discussed within and that any recommendations or suggestions that are made herein are for entertainment purposes only. Professionals should be consulted as needed prior to undertaking any of the action endorsed herein.

This declaration is deemed fair and valid by both the American Bar Association and the Committee of Publishers Association and is legally binding throughout the United States. Furthermore, the transmission, duplication, or reproduction of any of the following work including specific information will be considered an illegal act irrespective of if it is done electronically or in print. This extends to creating a secondary or tertiary copy of the work or a recorded copy and is only allowed with the express written consent from the Publisher. All additional right reserved.

The information in the following pages is broadly considered a truthful and accurate account of facts and as such, any inattention, use, or misuse of the information in question by the reader will render any resulting actions solely under their purview. There are no scenarios in which the publisher or the original author of this work can be in any fashion deemed liable for any hardship or damages that may befall them after undertaking information described herein.

Additionally, the information in the following pages is intended only for informational purposes and should thus be thought of as universal. As befitting its nature, it is presented without assurance regarding its prolonged validity or interim quality. Trademarks that are mentioned are done without written consent and can in no way be considered an endorsement from the trademark holder.

Introduction

A Keto diet for vegetarians, is focused on proportionately eating more foods primarily from plants and cutting back on animal-derived foods. However, it does not necessarily involve eliminating entire food groups and lean sources of protein. This means, those on a plant-based diet may still opt to eat some meat.

Going vegan, on the other hand, means being strictly against animal products in any form—from never eating meat and dairy products to not patronizing products tested on animals and not wearing animal products such as leather.

A healthy plant-based diet generally emphasizes meeting your nutritional needs by eating more whole plant foods, while reducing the intake of animal products. Whole foods refer to natural, unrefined or minimally refined foods. Plant foods consist of those that do not have animal ingredients such as meat, eggs, honey, milk and other dairy products.

In contrast, those on a vegetarian diet may still eat processed and refined foods. Vegetarians can even eat fast foods, junk food and other salty snacks guilt-free. Once you get started with this diet, you will notice a huge difference in how you feel each day. From the time that you wake up in the morning, you will feel that you have more energy, and that you do not get tired as easily as before. You will also have more mental focus and fewer mood-related problems.

As for digestion, a plant-based diet is also said to improve how the digestive system works. In fact, dieters confirm fewer incidences of stomach pains, bloating, indigestion and hyperacidity.

Then there's the weight loss benefit that we cannot forget about. Since a plant-based diet means eating fruits, vegetables, and whole grains that have fewer calories and are lower in fat, you will enjoy weight loss benefits that some other fad diets are not able to provide.

Aside from helping you lose weight; it maintains ideal weight longer because this diet is easier to sustain and does not require elimination of certain food groups.

Don't worry about not getting enough nutrients from your food intake. This diet provides all the necessary nutrients including proteins, vitamins, minerals, carbohydrates, fats, and antioxidants. And again, that's because it does not eliminate any food group but only encourages you to focus more on plant-based food products.

As you can imagine, humans have been consuming a plant-based diet before the invention of McDonald's and some of our other favorite fast-food chains. To begin our journey, I am going to start us off in the times of the hunter-gatherer. While we could go back even further (think Ancient Egypt!), I believe this is where a plant-based diet becomes most relevant.

The hunter-gatherer time period is where we find the earliest evidence of hunting. While we do have a long history of eating meat, this was a point in time where consuming meat was very limited. Of course, humans eating meat does not mean we were carnivores; in fact, the way we are built tells us differently. Yes, we can consume meat, but humans are considered omnivores. You can tell this from our jaw design, running speeds, alimentary tract, and the fact we don't have claws attached to our fingers. History also tells us we are omnivores by nature; however, the evolution of our human brains led us to become hunters so that we could survive.

The need for hunting did not come around until our ancestors left tropical regions. Other locations influenced the availability of plant-based foods. Instead of enduring winter with limited amounts of food, we had to adapt! Of course, out of hunger, animal-flesh becomes much more appealing. This early in time, our ancestors did not have a grocery store to just pop in and buy whatever they needed. Instead, they used the opportunity of hunting and gathering to keep themselves alive.

Eventually, we moved away from hunting and gathering and started to become farmers. While this timeline is a bit tricky and agricultural history began at different points in different parts of the world, all that matters is that at some point; animals started to become domesticated and dairy, eggs, and meat all became readily available. Once this started, humans no longer needed to hunt nor gather because the farmers provided everything we could desire

While starting a plant-based diet is an excellent idea and has many wonderful benefits let's be honest, you are mostly here to benefit yourself. It is fantastic that you are deciding to put you and your health first. You deserve to be the best version of yourself, with a little bit of legwork, you will be there in no time

To some people, a plant-based diet is just another fad diet. There are so many diets on the market right now, why is plant-based any different? Whether you are looking to lose weight, reverse disease, or just love animals.

A plant-based diet is so much more than just eating fruits and vegetables. This is a lifestyle where you are encouraged to journey to a better version of yourself. As you improve your eating habits, you will need something to do with all of your new found energy! It is time to gain control over your eating habits and figure out how food truly does affect our daily lives! Below, you will find the amazing benefits a plant-based diet has to offer you.

Breakfast

Pumpkin pancakes

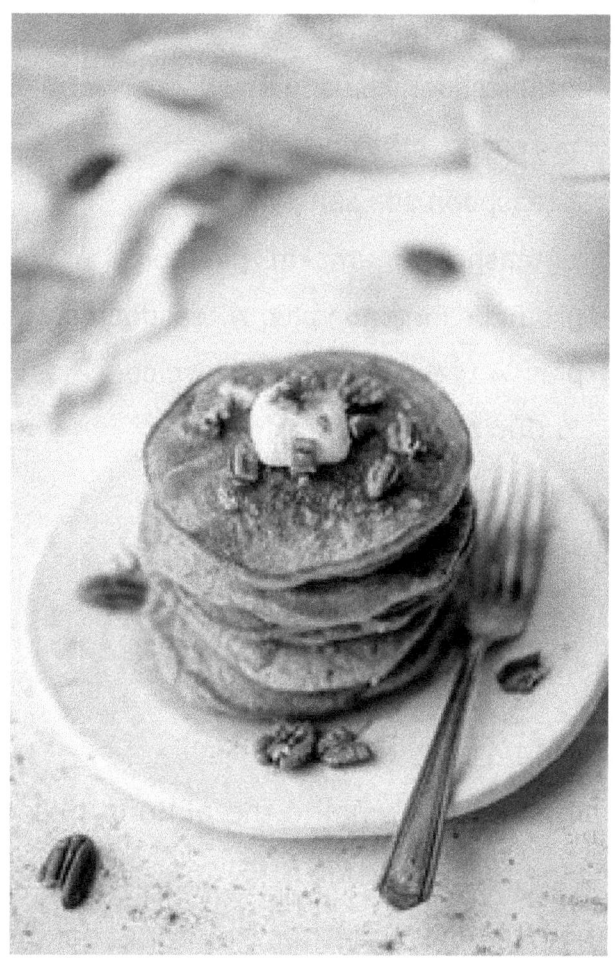

Preparation Time: 15 minutes

Cooking Time: 15 minutes

Servings: 4

Ingredients

- 2 cups unsweetened almond milk
- 1 teaspoon apple cider vinegar
- 2½ cups whole-wheat flour
- 2 tablespoons baking powder
- ½ Teaspoon baking soda
- 1 teaspoon sea salt
- 1 teaspoon pumpkin pie spice or ½ teaspoon ground -cinnamon plus ¼ teaspoon grated -nutmeg plus ¼ teaspoon ground allspice
- ½ Cup canned pumpkin purée
- 1 cup water
- 1 tablespoon coconut oil

Directions

In a small bowl, combine the almond milk and apple cider vinegar. Set aside.

In a bowl, whisk together the flour, baking powder, baking soda, salt, and pumpkin pie spice. In bowl, combine the almond milk mixture, pumpkin purée, and water, whisking to mix well. Mix the wet Ingredients to the dry Ingredients and fold together until the dry -Ingredients are just moistened.

In a nonstick pan or griddle over medium-high heat, melt the coconut oil and swirl to coat. Pour the batter into the pan ¼ cup at a time and cook until the pancakes are browned, about 5 minutes per side. Serve immediately.

Nutrition

- calories 270
- fat 15,
- fiber 3
- carbs 5
- protein 9

Quinoa Applesauce Muffins

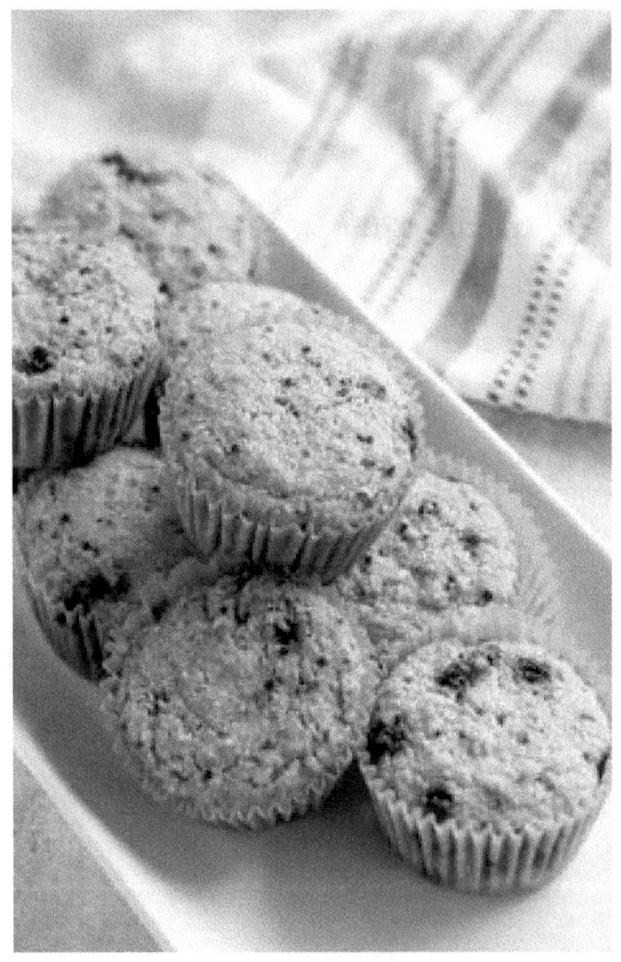

Preparation Time: 10 minutes

Cooking Time: 15 minutes

Servings: 5

Ingredients

2 tablespoons coconut oil or margarine, melted, plus more for coating the muffin tin

¼ Cup ground flaxseed

½ Cup water

2 cups unsweetened applesauce

½ Cup brown sugar

1 teaspoon apple cider vinegar

2½ cups whole-grain flour

1½ cups cooked quinoa

2 teaspoons baking soda

Pinch salt

½ Cup dried cranberries or raisins

Directions

Preheat the oven to 400°f.

Coat a muffin tin with coconut oil, line with paper muffin cups, or use a nonstick tin. In a large bowl, stir together the flaxseed and water. Add the applesauce, sugar, coconut oil, and vinegar. Stir to combine. Add the flour, quinoa, baking soda, and salt, stirring until just combined. Gently fold in the cranberries without stirring too much. Scoop the muffin mixture into the prepared tin, about ⅓ cup for each muffin.

Bake for 15 to 20 minutes, until slightly browned on top and springy to the touch. Let cool for about 10 minutes. Run a dinner knife around the inside of each cup to loosen, then tilt the muffins on their sides in the muffin wells so air gets underneath. These keep in an airtight container in the refrigerator for up to 1 week or in the freezer indefinitely.

Nutrition

calories: 387

protein: 7g

total fat: 5g

saturated fat: 2g

carbohydrates: 57g

fiber: 8g

Green breakfast smoothie

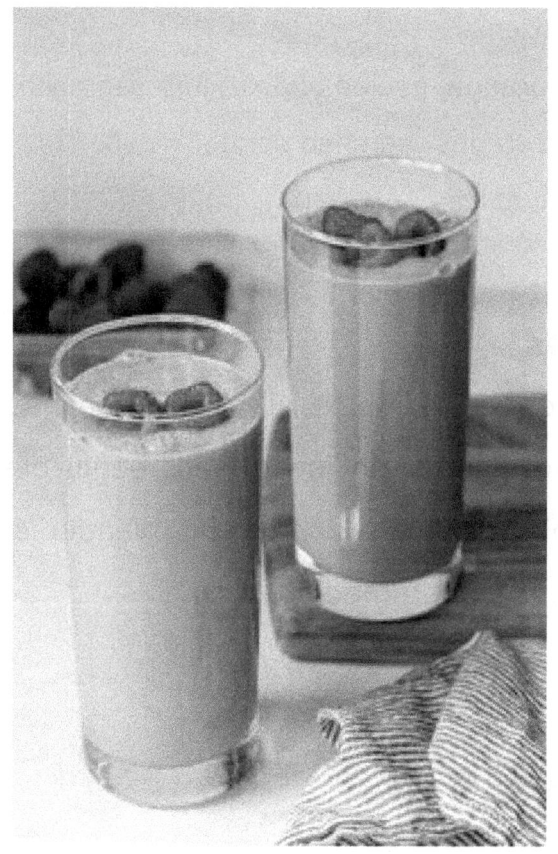

Preparation Time: 10 minutes

Cooking Time: 0 minutes

Servings: 2

Ingredients

- ½ Banana, sliced
- 2 cups spinach or other greens, such as kale
- 1 cup sliced berries of your choosing, fresh or frozen
- 1 orange, peeled and cut into segments
- 1 cup unsweetened nondairy milk
- 1 cup ice

Directions

In a blender, combine all the Ingredients. Starting with the blender on low speed, begin blending the smoothie, gradually increasing blender speed until smooth. Serve immediately.

Nutrition

calories 270

fat 15

fiber 3

carbs 5

protein 9

Blueberry Lemonade Smoothie

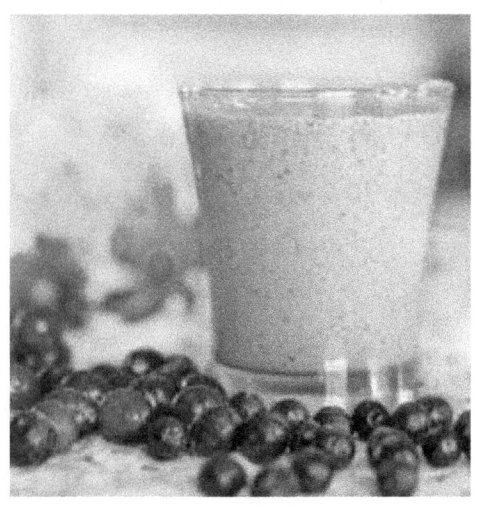

Preparation Time : 10 minutes

Cooking Time: 10 minutes

Servings: 1

Ingredients

- 1 cup roughly chopped kale
- ¾ Cup frozen blueberries
- 1 cup unsweetened soy or almond milk
- Juice of 1 lemon

- 1 tablespoon maple syrup

Directions

Combine all the Ingredients in a blender and blend until smooth. Enjoy immediately.

Nutrition
- Calories; 398
- Fat 21g
- Carbs 4.7g
- Proteins 44.2g
- Sugars 0.5g

Berry Protein Smoothie

Preparation Time: 5 minutes

Cooking Time: 0 minutes

Servings: 1

Ingredients

- 1 banana
- 1 cup fresh or frozen berries
- ¾ Cup water or nondairy milk, plus more as needed
- 1 scoop plant-based protein powder, 3 ounces silken tofu, ¼ cup rolled oats, or ½ cup cooked quinoa
- Additions
- 1 tablespoon ground flaxseed or chia seeds
- 1 handful fresh spinach or lettuce, or 1 chunk cucumber
- Coconut water to replace some of the liquid

Directions

In a blender, combine the banana, berries, water,

and your choice of protein.

Add any addition Ingredients as desired. Purée until smooth and creamy, about 50 seconds.

Add a bit more water if you like a thinner smoothie.

Nutrition
- calories: 332
- protein: 7g
- total fat: 5g
- saturated fat: 1g
- carbohydrates: 72g
- fiber: 11g

Almond Plum Oats Overnight

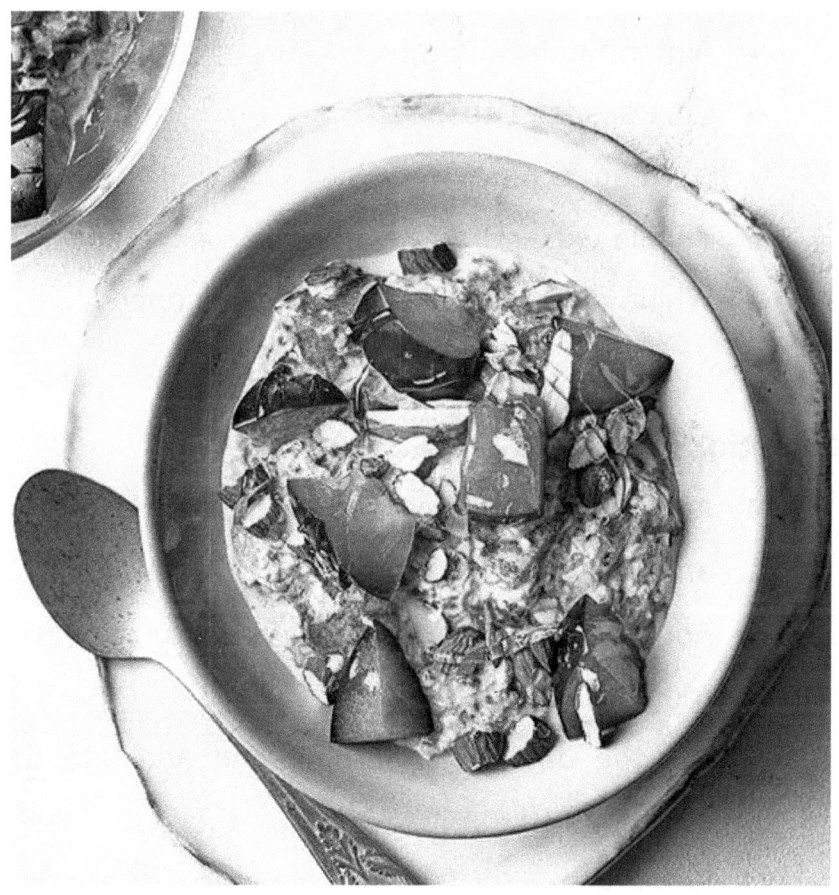

Preparation Time: 10 minutes

Cooking Time: 10 minutes plus overnight

Servings: 2

Ingredients
- Rolled oats: 60g
- Plums: 3 ripe and chopped
- Almond milk: 300ml
- Chia seeds: 1 tbsp
- Nutmeg: a pinch
- Vanilla extract: a few drops
- Whole almonds: 1 tbsp roughly chopped

Directions:
1. Add oats, nutmeg, vanilla extract, almond milk, and chia seeds to a bowl and mix well
2. Add in cubed plums and cover and place in the fridge for a night
3. Mix the oats well morning and add into the serving bowl
4. Serve with your favorite toppings

Nutrition
- Carbs: 24.7g

- Protein: 9.5g
- Fats: 10.8g
- Calories: 248Kcal

Avocado Miso Chickpeas Toast

Preparation Time: 10 minutes
Cooking Time: 15 minutes
Servings: 2

Ingredients

- Chickpeas: 400g drained and rinsed
- Avocado: 1 medium
- Toasted sesame oil: 1 tsp
- White miso paste: 1 ½ tbsp
- Sesame seeds: 1 tbsp
- Spring onion: 1 finely sliced
- Lemon:1 half for the juice and half wedged to serve
- Rye bread: 4 slices toasted

Directions:

1. In a bowl add sesame oil, chickpeas, miso, and lemon juice and mash using a potato masher

2. Roughly crushed avocado in another bowl using a fork
3. Add the avocado to the chickpeas and make a spread
4. Spread it on a toast and top with spring onion and sesame seeds
5. Serve with lemon wedges

Nutrition
- Carbs: 33.3 g
- Protein: 14.6 g
- Fats: 26.6 g
- Calories: 456 Kcal

Banana Malt Bread

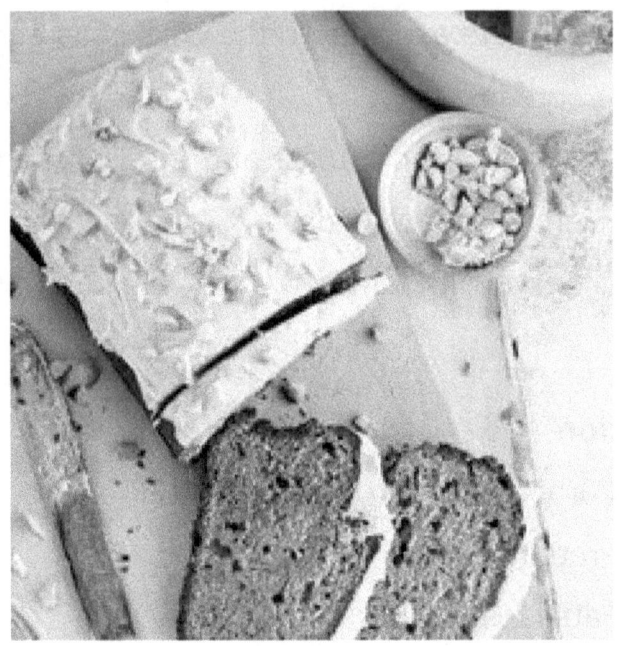

Preparation Time: 10 minutes

Cooking Time: 1 hour 20 minutes and Maturing Time

Servings: 12 slices

Ingredients

- Hot strong black tea: 120ml
- Malt extract: 150g plus extra for brushing
- Bananas:2 ripe mashed
- Sultanas: 100g
- Pitted dates:120g chopped

- Plain flour: 250g
- Soft dark brown sugar: 50g
- Baking powder: 2 tsp

Directions:
1. Preheat the oven to 140C
2. Line the loaf tin with the baking paper
3. Brew tea and include sultanas and dates to it
4. Take a small pan and heat the malt extract and gradually add sugar to it
5. Stir continuously and let it cook
6. In a bowl, add flour, salt, and baking powder and now top with sugar extract, fruits, bananas, and tea
7. Mix the batter well and add to the loaf tin
8. Bake the mixture for an hour
9. Brush the bread with extra malt extract and let it cool down before removing from the tin
10. When done, wrap in a foil; it can be consumed for a week

Nutrition

- Carbs: 43.3 g
- Protein: 3.4 g
- Fats: 0.3 g
- Calories: 194 Kcal

Banana Vegan Bread

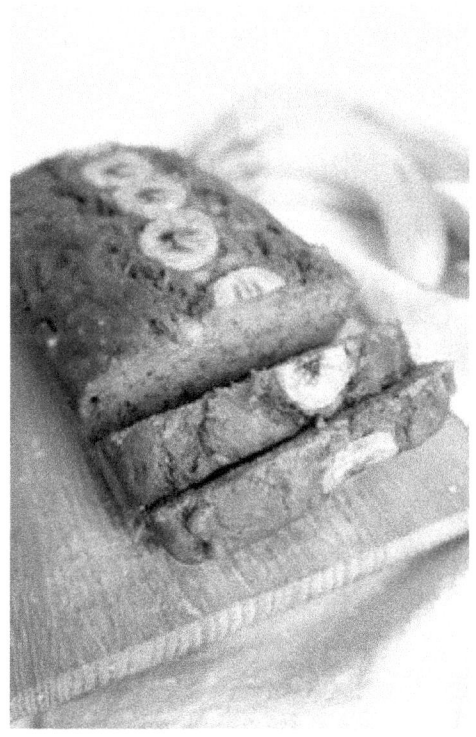

Preparation Time: 15 minutes

Cooking Time: 1 hour 15 minutes

Servings: 1 loaf

Ingredients

- Overripe banana: 3 large mashed
- All-purpose flour: 200 g

- Unsweetened non-dairy milk: 50 ml
- White vinegar: ½ tsp
- Ground flaxseed: 10 g
- Ground cinnamon: ¼ tsp
- Granulated sugar: 140 g
- Vanilla: ¼ tsp
- Baking powder: ¼ tsp
- Baking soda: ¼ tsp
- Salt: ¼ tsp
- Canola oil: 3 tbsp
- Chopped walnuts: ½ cup

Directions:
1. Preheat the oven to 350F and line the loaf pan with parchment paper
2. Mash bananas using a fork
3. Take a large bowl, and add in mash bananas, canola oil, oat milk, sugar, vinegar, vanilla, and ground flax seed
4. Also whisk in baking powder, cinnamon, flour, and salt
5. Add batter to the loaf pan and bake for 50 minutes

6. Remove from pan and let it sit for 10 minutes
7. Slice when completely cooled down

Nutrition
- Carbs: 40.3g
- Protein: 2.8g
- Fats: 8.2g
- Calories: 240Kcal

Berry Compote Pancakes

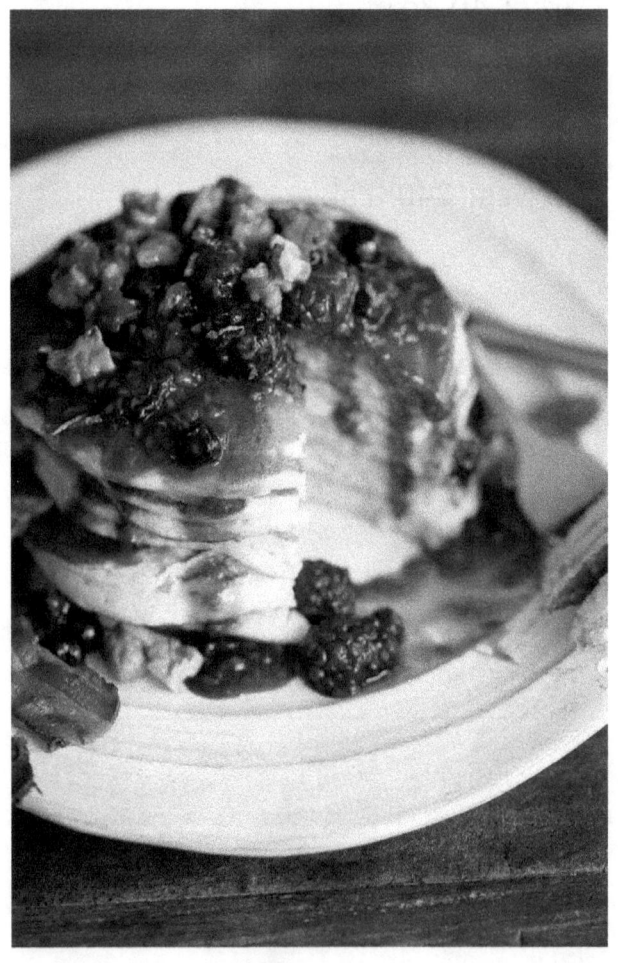

Preparation Time: 5 minutes

Cooking Time: 30 minutes

Servings: 2

Ingredients

- Mixed frozen berries: 200g
- Plain flour: 140 g
- Unsweetened almond milk: 140ml
- Icing sugar: 1 tbsp
- Lemon juice: 1 tbsp
- Baking powder: 2 tsp
- Vanilla extract: a dash
- Salt: a pinch
- Caster sugar: 2 tbsp
- Vegetable oil: ½ tbsp

Directions:

1. Take a small pan and add berries, lemon juice, and icing sugar
2. Cook the mixture for 10 minutes to give it a saucy texture and set aside
3. Take a bowl and add caster sugar, flour, baking powder, and salt and mix well

4. Add in almond milk and vanilla and combine well to make a batter
5. Take a non-stick pan, and heat 2 teaspoons oil in it and spread it over the whole surface
6. Add ¼ cup of the batter to the pan and cook each side for 3-4 minutes
7. Serve with compote

Nutrition
- Carbs: 92 g
- Protein: 9.4 g
- Fats: 5.2 g
- Calories: 463 Kcal

Buckwheat Crepes

Preparation Time: 15 minutes

Cooking Time: 25 minutes

Servings: 12

Ingredients

- Raw buckwheat flour: 1 cup
- Light coconut milk: 1 and 3/4 cups
- Ground cinnamon: 1/8 tsp
- Flaxseeds: 3/4 tbsp
- Melted coconut oil: 1 tbsp
- Sea salt: a pinch
- Any sweetener: as per your taste

Directions:

1. Take a bowl and add flaxseed, coconut milk, salt, avocado, and cinnamon
2. Mix them all well and fold in the flour
3. Now take a nonstick pan and pour oil and provide gentle heat
4. Add a big spoon of a mixture
5. Cook till it appears bubbly, then change side

6. Perform the task until all crepes are prepared
7. For enhancing the taste, add the sweetener of your liking

Nutrition

Carbs: 8g

Protein: 1g

Fats: 3g

Calories: 71Kcal

Chickpeas Spread Sourdough Toast

Preparation Time: 15 minutes

Cooking Time: 15 minutes

Servings: 4

Ingredients

- Chickpeas: 1 cup rinsed and drained
- Pumpkin puree: 1 cup
- Vegan yogurt: ½ cup
- Salt: as per your need
- Sourdough: 4 slices toasted

Directions:

1. In a bowl add chickpeas and pumpkin puree and mash using a potato masher
2. Add in salt and yogurt and mix
3. Spread it on a toast and serve

Nutrition
- Carbs: 33.7g
- Protein: 8.45g
- Fats: 2.5g
- Calories: 187Kcal

Chickpeas with Harissa

Preparation Time: 15 minutes

Cooking Time: 20 minutes

Servings: 2

Ingredients

- Chickpeas: 1 cup can rinse and drained well
- Onion: 1 small diced
- Cucumber: 1 cup diced
- Tomato: 1 cup diced
- Salt: as per your taste
- Lemon juice: 2 tbsp
- Harissa: 2 tsp
- Olive oil: 1 tbsp
- Flat-leaf parsley: 2 tbsp chopped

Directions:

1. Add lemon juice, harissa, and olive oil in a bowl and whisk

2. Take a serving bowl and add onion, cucumber, chickpeas, salt and the sauce you made
3. Add parsley from the top and serve

Nutrition
- Carbs: 55.6 g
- Protein: 17.8g
- Fats: 11.8g
- Calories: 398Kcal

Lunch

Whipped Potatoes

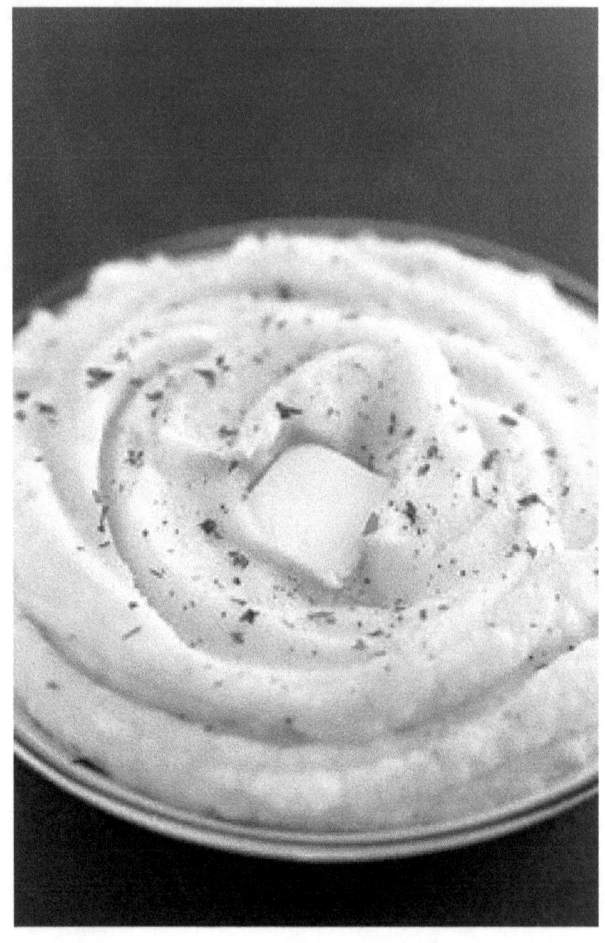

Preparation Time: 20 minutes

Cooking Time: 35 minutes

Servings: 10

Ingredients

- 4 cups water
- 3 lb. potatoes, sliced into cubes
- 3 cloves garlic, crushed
- 6 tablespoons butter
- 2 bay leaves
- 10 sage leaves
- ½ cup Greek yogurt
- ¼ cup low-fat milk
- Salt to taste

Direction

1. Boil the potatoes in water for 30 minutes or until tender.
2. Drain.
3. In a pan over medium heat, cook the garlic in butter for 1 minute.
4. Add the sage and cook for 5 more minutes.
5. Discard the garlic.
6. Use a fork to mash the potatoes.
7. Whip using an electric mixer while gradually adding the butter, yogurt, and milk.
8. Season with salt.

Nutrition

- Calories: 169
- Total fat: 7.6g
- Saturated fat: 4.7g
- Cholesterol: 21mg
- Sodium: 251mg

Quinoa Avocado Salad

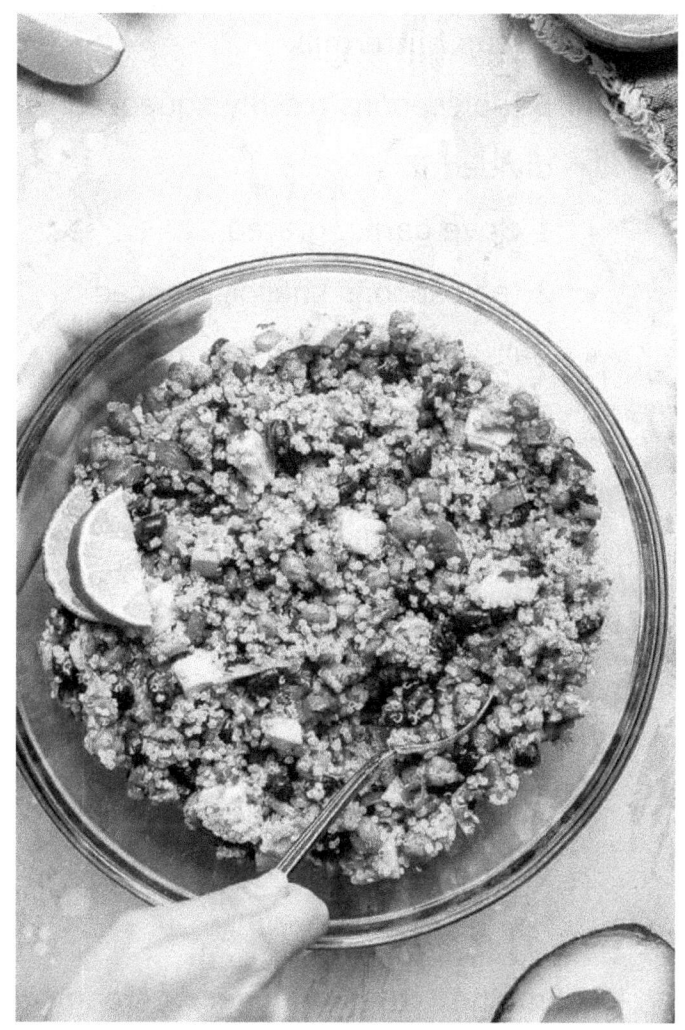

Preparation Time: 15 minutes

Cooking Time: 4 minutes

Servings: 4

Ingredients

- 2 tablespoons balsamic vinegar
- ¼ cup cream
- ¼ cup buttermilk
- 5 tablespoons freshly squeezed lemon juice, divided
- 1 clove garlic, grated
- 2 tablespoons shallot, minced
- Salt and pepper to taste
- 2 tablespoons avocado oil, divided
- 1 ¼ cups quinoa, cooked
- 2 heads endive, sliced
- 2 firm pears, sliced thinly
- 2 avocados, sliced
- ¼ cup fresh dill, chopped

Direction

1. Combine the vinegar, cream, milk, 1 tablespoon lemon juice, garlic, shallot, salt and pepper in a bowl.
2. Pour 1 tablespoon oil into a pan over medium heat.

3. Heat the quinoa for 4 minutes.
4. Transfer quinoa to a plate.
5. Toss the endive and pears in a mixture of remaining oil, remaining lemon juice, salt and pepper.
6. Transfer to a plate.
7. Toss the avocado in the reserved dressing.
8. Add to the plate.
9. Top with the dill and quinoa.

Nutrition

- Calories: 431
- Total fat: 28.5g
- Saturated fat: 8g
- Cholesterol: 13mg

Roasted Sweet Potatoes

Preparation Time: 20 minutes

Cooking Time: 20 minutes

Servings: 4

Ingredients:

- 2 potatoes, sliced into wedges
- 2 tablespoons olive oil, divided
- Salt and pepper to taste
- 1 red bell pepper, chopped
- ¼ cup fresh cilantro, chopped
- 1 garlic, minced
- 2 tablespoons almonds, toasted and sliced
- 1 tablespoon lime juice

Direction:

1. Preheat your oven to 425 degrees F.
2. Toss the sweet potatoes in oil and salt.
3. Transfer to a baking pan.
4. Roast for 20 minutes.

5. In a bowl, combine the red bell pepper, cilantro, garlic and almonds.
6. In another bowl, mix the lime juice, remaining oil, salt and pepper.
7. Drizzle this mixture over the red bell pepper mixture.
8. Serve sweet potatoes with the red bell pepper mixture.

Nutrition
- Calories: 146
- Total fat: 8.6g
- Saturated fat: 1.1g
- Sodium: 317mg

Cauliflower Salad

Preparation Time: 20 minutes

Cooking Time: 15 minutes

Servings: 4

Ingredients:

- 8 cups cauliflower florets
- 5 tablespoons olive oil, divided
- Salt and pepper to taste
- 1 cup parsley
- 1 clove garlic, minced
- 2 tablespoons lemon juice
- ¼ cup almonds, toasted and sliced
- 3 cups arugula
- 2 tablespoons olives, sliced
- ¼ cup feta, crumbled

Direction

1. Preheat your oven to 425 degrees F.
2. Toss the cauliflower in a mixture of 1 tablespoon olive oil, salt and pepper.

3. Place in a baking pan and roast for 15 minutes.
4. Put the parsley, remaining oil, garlic, lemon juice, salt and pepper in a blender.
5. Pulse until smooth.
6. Place the roasted cauliflower in a salad bowl.
7. Stir in the rest of the ingredients along with the parsley dressing.

Nutrition
- Calories: 198
- Total fat: 16.5g
- Saturated fat: 3g
- Cholesterol: 6mg

Garlic Mashed Potatoes & Turnips

Preparation Time: 20 minutes

Cooking Time: 30 minutes

Servings: 8

Ingredients:

- 1 head garlic
- 1 teaspoon olive oil
- 1 lb. turnips, sliced into cubes
- 2 lb. potatoes, sliced into cubes
- ½ cup almond milk
- ½ cup Parmesan cheese, grated
- 1 tablespoon fresh thyme, chopped
- 1 tablespoon fresh chives, chopped
- 2 tablespoons butter
- Salt and pepper to taste

Direction:

1. Preheat your oven to 375 degrees F.

2. Slice the tip off the garlic head.
3. Drizzle with a little oil and roast in the oven for 45 minutes.
4. Boil the turnips and potatoes in a pot of water for 30 minutes or until tender.
5. Add all the ingredients to a food processor along with the garlic.
6. Pulse until smooth.

Nutrition

- Calories: 141
- Total fat: 3.2g
- Saturated fat: 1.5g
- Cholesterol: 7mg

Cashew Siam Salad

Preparation Time: 10 minutes

Cooking Time:: 3 minutes

Servings: 4

Ingredients:

Salad:

- 4 cups baby spinach, rinsed, drained
- ½ cup pickled red cabbage

Dressing:

- 1-inch piece ginger, finely chopped
- 1 tsp. chili garlic paste
- 1 tbsp. soy sauce
- ½ tbsp. rice vinegar
- 1 tbsp. sesame oil
- 3 tbsp. avocado oil

Toppings:

- ½ cup raw cashews, unsalted
- ¼ cup fresh cilantro, chopped

Directions:

1. Put the spinach and red cabbage in a large bowl. Toss to combine and set the salad aside.
2. Toast the cashews in a frying pan over medium-high heat, stirring occasionally until the cashews are golden brown. This should take about 3 minutes. Turn off the heat and set the frying pan aside.
3. Mix all the dressing ingredients in a medium-sized bowl and use a spoon to mix them into a smooth dressing.
4. Pour the dressing over the spinach salad and top with the toasted cashews.
5. Toss the salad to combine all ingredients and transfer the large bowl to the fridge. Allow the salad to chill for up to one hour – doing so will guarantee a better flavor. Alternatively, the salad can be served right away, topped with the optional cilantro. Enjoy!

Nutrition:

- Calories 236
- Carbohydrates 6.1 g

- Fats 21.6 g
- Protein 4.2 g

Avocado and Cauliflower Hummus

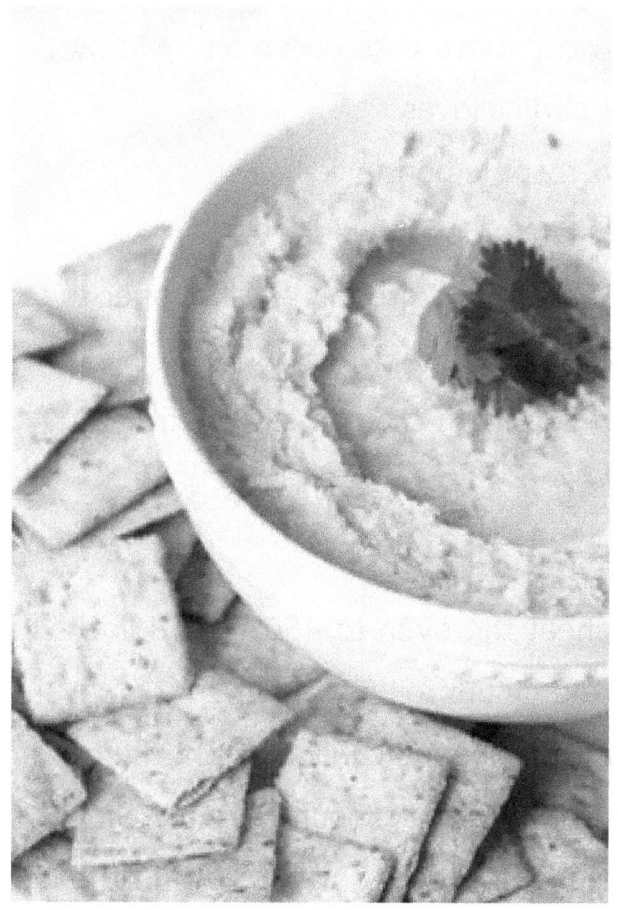

Preparation Time: 5 minutes

Cooking Time:: 25 minutes

Servings: 2

Ingredients:

- 1 medium cauliflower, stem removed and chopped
- 1 large Hass avocado, peeled, pitted, and chopped
- ¼ cup extra virgin olive oil
- 2 garlic cloves
- ½ tbsp. lemon juice
- ½ tsp. onion powder
- Sea salt and ground black pepper to taste
- 2 large carrots
- ¼ cup fresh cilantro, chopped

Directions:

1. Preheat the oven to 450°F, and line a baking tray with aluminum foil.
2. Put the chopped cauliflower on the baking tray and drizzle with 2 tablespoons of olive oil.
3. Roast the chopped cauliflower in the oven for 20-25 minutes, until lightly brown.
4. Remove the tray from the oven and allow the cauliflower to cool down.
5. Add all the ingredients—except the carrots and

optional fresh cilantro—to a food processor or blender, and blend the ingredients into a smooth hummus.

6.Transfer the hummus to a medium-sized bowl, cover, and put it in the fridge for at least 30 minutes.

7.Take the hummus out of the fridge and, if desired, top it with the optional chopped cilantro and more salt and pepper to taste; serve with the carrot fries, and enjoy!

Nutrition:

- Calories 416
- Carbohydrates 8.4 g
- Fats 40.3 g
- Protein 3.3 g

Raw Zoodles with Avocado 'N Nuts

Preparation Time: 10 minutes

Servings: 2

Ingredients:

- 1 medium zucchini
- 1½ cups basil
- 1/3 cup water
- 5 tbsp. pine nuts
- 2 tbsp. lemon juice
- 1 medium avocado, peeled, pitted, sliced
- Optional: 2 tbsp. olive oil
- 6 yellow cherry tomatoes, halved
- Optional: 6 red cherry tomatoes, halved
- Sea salt and black pepper to taste

Directions:

1. Add the basil, water, nuts, lemon juice, avocado slices, optional olive oil (if desired), salt, and pepper to a blender.

2. Blend the ingredients into a smooth mixture. Add more salt and pepper to taste and blend again.

3. Divide the sauce and the zucchini noodles between two medium-sized bowls for serving, and combine in each.

4. Top the mixtures with the halved yellow cherry tomatoes, and the optional red cherry tomatoes (if desired); serve and enjoy!

Nutrition:
- Calories 317
- Carbohydrates 7.4 g
- Fats 28.1 g
- Protein 7.2 g

Cauliflower Sushi

Preparation Time: 30 minutes

Servings: 4

Ingredients:

Sushi Base:

- 6 cups cauliflower florets
- ½ cup vegan cheese
- 1 medium spring onion, diced
- 4 nori sheets
- Sea salt and pepper to taste
- 1 tbsp. rice vinegar or sushi vinegar
- 1 medium garlic clove, minced

Filling:

- 1 medium Hass avocado, peeled, sliced
- ½ medium cucumber, skinned, sliced
- 4 asparagus spears
- A handful of enoki mushrooms

Directions:

1. Put the cauliflower florets in a food processor or

blender. Pulse the florets into a rice-like substance. When using readymade cauliflower rice, add this to the blender.

2.Add the vegan cheese, spring onions, and vinegar to the food processor or blender. Top these ingredients with salt and pepper to taste, and pulse everything into a chunky mixture. Make sure not to turn the ingredients into a puree by pulsing too long.

3.Taste and add more vinegar, salt, or pepper to taste. Add the optional minced garlic clove to the blender and pulse again for a few seconds.

4.Lay out the nori sheets and spread the cauliflower rice mixture out evenly between the sheets. Make sure to leave at least 2 inches of the top and bottom edges empty.

5.Place one or more combinations of multiple filling ingredients along the center of the spread out rice mixture. Experiment with different ingredients per nori sheet for the best flavor.

6.Roll up each nori sheet tightly. (Using a sushi mat will make this easier.)

7.Either serve the sushi as a nori roll, or, slice each roll up into sushi pieces.

8. Serve right away with a small amount of wasabi, pickled ginger, and soy sauce!

Nutrition:
- Calories 189
- Carbohydrates 7.6 g
- Fats 14.4 g
- Protein 6.1 g

Spinach and Mashed Tofu Salad

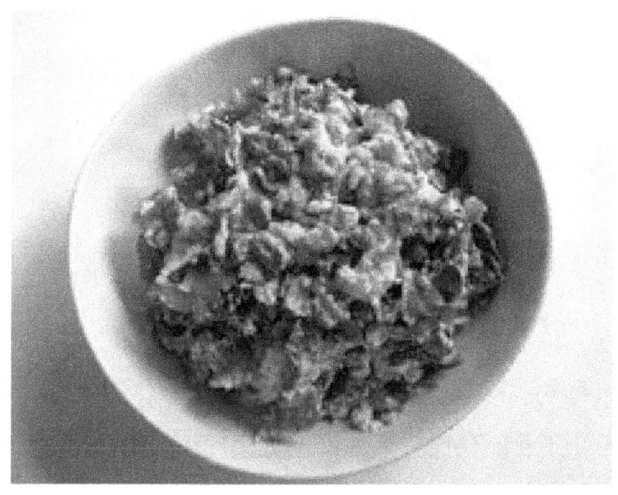

Preparation Time: 20 minutes

Cooking Time: 15 minutes

Servings: 4

Ingredients:

- 2 8-oz. blocks firm tofu, drained
- 4 cups baby spinach leaves
- 4 tbsp. cashew butter
- 1½ tbsp. soy sauce

- 1-inch piece ginger, finely chopped
- 1 tsp. red miso paste
- 2 tbsp. sesame seeds
- 1 tsp. organic orange zest
- 1 tsp. nori flakes
- 2 tbsp. water

Directions:

1. Use paper towels to absorb any excess water left in the tofu before crumbling both blocks into small pieces.
2. In a large bowl, combine the mashed tofu with the spinach leaves.
3. Mix the remaining ingredients in another small bowl and, if desired, add the optional water for a more smooth dressing.
4. Pour this dressing over the mashed tofu and spinach leaves.
5. Transfer the bowl to the fridge and allow the salad to chill for up to one hour. Doing so will guarantee a better flavor. Or, the salad can be served right away. Enjoy!

Nutrition:

- Calories 166
- Carbohydrates 5.5 g
- Fats 10.7 g
- Protein 11.3 g

Cucumber Edamame Salad

Preparation Time: 5 minutes

Cooking Time:: 8 minutes

Servings: 2

Ingredients:

- 3 tbsp. avocado oil
- 1 cup cucumber, sliced into thin rounds
- ½ cup fresh sugar snap peas, sliced or whole
- ½ cup fresh edamame
- ¼ cup radish, sliced
- 1 large Hass avocado, peeled, pitted, sliced
- 1 nori sheet, crumbled
- 2 tsp. roasted sesame seeds
- 1 tsp. salt

Directions:

1. Bring a medium-sized pot filled halfway with water to a boil over medium-high heat.
2. Add the sugar snaps and cook them for about 2

minutes.

3. Take the pot off the heat, drain the excess water, transfer the sugar snaps to a medium-sized bowl and set aside for now.

4. Fill the pot with water again, add the teaspoon of salt and bring to a boil over medium-high heat.

5. Add the edamame to the pot and let them cook for about 6 minutes.

6. Take the pot off the heat, drain the excess water, transfer the soybeans to the bowl with sugar snaps and let them cool down for about 5 minutes.

7. Combine all ingredients, except the nori crumbs and roasted sesame seeds, in a medium-sized bowl.

8. Carefully stir, using a spoon, until all ingredients are evenly coated in oil.

9. Top the salad with the nori crumbs and roasted sesame seeds.

10. Transfer the bowl to the fridge and allow the salad to cool for at least 30 minutes.

11. Serve chilled and enjoy!

Nutrition:
- Calories 409

- Carbohydrates 7.1 g
- Fats 38.25 g
- Protein 7.6 g

Artichoke White Bean Sandwich Spread

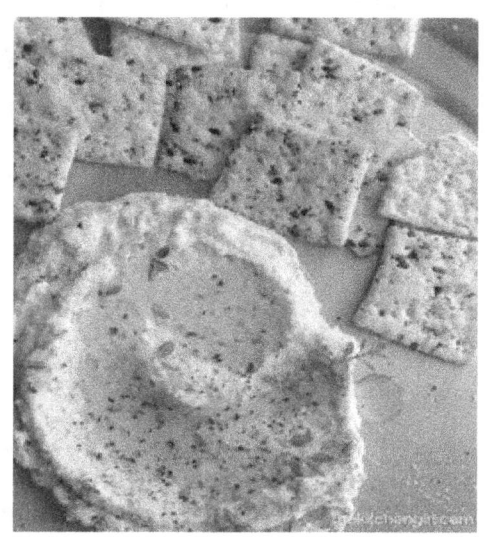

Preparation Time: 10 minutes

Cooking Time: 15 minutes

Servings: 2

Ingredients:

- ½ cup raw cashews, chopped
- Water
- 1 clove garlic, cut into half

- 1 tablespoon lemon zest
- 1 teaspoon fresh rosemary, chopped
- ¼ teaspoon salt
- ¼ teaspoon pepper
- 6 tablespoons almond, soy or coconut milk
- 1 15.5-ounce can cannellini beans, rinsed and drained well
- 3 to 4 canned artichoke hearts, chopped
- ¼ cup hulled sunflower seeds
- Green onions, chopped, for garnish

Directions:

1. Soak the raw cashews for 15 minutes in enough water to cover them. Drain and dab with a paper towel to make them as dry as possible.

2. Transfer the cashews to a blender and add the garlic, lemon zest, rosemary, salt and pepper. Pulse to break everything up and then add the milk, one tablespoon at a time, until the mixture is smooth and creamy.

3. Mash the beans in a bowl with a fork. Add the artichoke hearts and sunflower seeds. Toss to mix.

4. Pour the cashew mixture on top and season with

more salt and pepper if desired. Mix the ingredients well and spread on whole-wheat bread, crackers, or a wrap.

Nutrition:
- Calories 110
- Carbohydrates 14 g
- Fats 4 g
- Protein 6 g

Dinner

Curried Tofu with Buttery Cabbage

Preparation Time: 15 minutes

Cooking Time: 10 minutes

Servings: 4

Ingredients

- 2 cups extra-firm tofu, pressed and cubed
- 1 tbsp + 3 ½ tbsp coconut oil
- ½ cup unsweetened shredded coconut
- 1 tsp yellow curry powder
- 1 tsp salt
- ½ tsp onion powder
- 2 cups Napa cabbage
- 4 oz. vegan butter
- Salt and black pepper to taste
- Lemon wedges for serving

Directions

1. In a medium bowl, add the tofu, 1 tablespoon of coconut oil, curry powder, salt, and onion powder. Mix well until the tofu is well-coated with the spices.
2. Heat the remaining coconut oil in a non-stick skillet and fry the tofu until golden brown on all sides, 8 minutes. Divide onto serving plates and set aside for serving.
3. In another skillet, melt half of the vegan butter, and sauté the cabbage until slightly caramelized, 2 minutes. Season with salt, black pepper, and plate to the side of the tofu.
4. Melt the remaining vegan butter in the skillet and drizzle all over the cabbage. Serve warm.

Nutrition

- calories 270
- fat 15
- fiber 3
- carbs 5
- protein 9

Smoked Tempeh with Broccoli Fritters

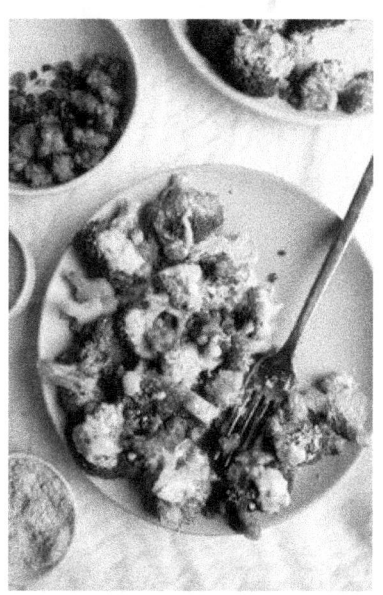

Preparation Time: 25 minutes

Cooking Time: 20 minutes

Servings: 4

Ingredients:

For the flax egg:
  4 tbsp flax seed powder + 12 tbsp water

For the grilled tempeh:

- 3 tbsp olive oil
- 1 tbsp soy sauce
- 3 tbsp fresh lime juice
- 1 tbsp grated ginger
- Salt and cayenne pepper to taste
- 10 oz. tempeh slices

For the broccoli fritters:
- 2 cups of rice broccoli
- 8 oz. tofu cheese
- 3 tbsp plain flour
- ½ tsp onion powder
- 1 tsp salt
- ¼ tsp freshly ground black pepper
- 4¼ oz. vegan butter

For serving:
- ½ cup mixed salad greens
- 1 cup vegan mayonnaise
- ½ lemon, juiced

Directions:
1. For the smoked tempeh:
2. In a bowl, mix the flax seed powder with water and set aside to soak for 5 minutes.
3. In another bowl, combine the olive oil, soy sauce, lime juice, grated ginger, salt, and cayenne pepper. Brush the tempeh slices with the mixture.
4. Heat a grill pan over medium heat and grill the tempeh on both sides until nicely smoked and golden brown, 8 minutes. Transfer to a plate and set aside in a warmer for serving.
5. In a medium bowl, combine the broccoli rice, tofu cheese, flour, onion, salt, and black pepper. Mix in the flax egg until well combine and form 1-inch thick patties out of the mixture.
6. Melt the vegan butter in a medium skillet over medium heat and fry the patties on both sides until golden brown, 8 minutes. Remove the fritters onto a plate and set aside.
7. In a small bowl, mix the vegan mayonnaise with the lemon juice.

8. Divide the smoked tempeh and broccoli fritters onto serving plates, add the salad greens, and serve with the vegan mayonnaise sauce.

Nutrition
- Calories; 21g
- Fat; 4.7g
- Carbs; 44.2g
- Protein; 0
- 0.5g Sugars

Cheesy Potato Casserole

Preparation Time: 30 minutes

Cooking Time: 20 minutes

Servings: 4

Ingredients:
- 2 oz. vegan butter
- ½ cup celery stalks, finely chopped
- 1 white onion, finely chopped
- 1 green bell pepper, seeded and finely chopped
- Salt and black pepper to taste
- 2 cups peeled and chopped potatoes
- 1 cup vegan mayonnaise
- 4 oz. freshly shredded vegan Parmesan cheese
- 1 tsp red chili flakes

Directions:
1. Preheat the oven to 400 F and grease a baking dish with cooking spray.

2. Season the celery, onion, and bell pepper with salt and black pepper.
3. In a bowl, mix the potatoes, vegan mayonnaise, Parmesan cheese, and red chili flakes.
4. Pour the mixture into the baking dish, add the season vegetables, and mix well.
5. Bake in the oven until golden brown, about 20 minutes.
6. Remove the baked potato and serve warm with baby spinach.

Nutrition
- calories 277
- fat 17
- fiber 5
- carbs 8
- protein 10

Curry Mushroom Pie

Preparation Time: 65 minutes

Cooking Time: 1 hour

Servings: 4

Ingredients:

For the piecrust:
- 1 tbsp flax seed powder + 3 tbsp water
- ¾ cup plain flour
- 4 tbsp. chia seeds
- 4 tbsp almond flour
- 1 tbsp nutritional yeast
- 1 tsp baking powder
- 1 pinch salt
- 3 tbsp olive oil
- 4 tbsp water

For the filling:
- 1 cup chopped baby Bella mushrooms
- 1 cup vegan mayonnaise

- 3 tbsp + 9 tbsp water
- ½ red bell pepper, finely chopped
- 1 tsp curry powder
- ½ tsp paprika powder
- ½ tsp garlic powder
- ¼ tsp black pepper
- ½ cup coconut cream
- 1 ¼ cups shredded vegan Parmesan cheese

Directions:

1. In two separate bowls, mix the different portions of flaxseed powder with the respective quantity of water. Allow soaking for 5 minutes.
2. For the piecrust:
3. Preheat the oven to 350 F.
4. When the flax egg is ready, pour the smaller quantity into a food processor and pour in all the ingredients for the piecrust. Blend until soft, smooth dough forms.
5. Line an 8-inch springform pan with parchment paper and grease with cooking spray.
6. Spread the dough in the bottom of the pan and bake for 15 minutes.

7. For the filling:
8. In a bowl, add the remaining flax egg and all the filling's ingredients. Combine well and pour the mixture on the piecrust. Bake further for 40 minutes or until the pie is golden brown.
9. Remove from the oven and allow cooling for 1 minute.
10. Slice and serve the pie warm.

Nutrition
- Calories 210
- Fat 3.7g
- Carbs 49.2g
- Protein 0.5g

Spicy Cheesy Tofu Balls

Preparation Time: 30 minutes

Cooking Time: 15 minutes

Servings: 4

Ingredients:

- 1/3 cup vegan mayonnaise
- ¼ cup pickled jalapenos
- 1 pinch cayenne pepper
- 4 oz. grated vegan cheddar cheese
- 1 tsp paprika powder
- 1 tbsp mustard powder
- 1 tbsp flax seed powder + 3 tbsp water
- 2 ½ cup crumbled tofu
- Salt and black pepper to taste
- 2 tbsp vegan butter, for frying

Directions:

1. For the spicy cheese:

2. In a bowl, mix all the ingredients for the spicy vegan cheese until well combined. Set aside.
3. In another medium bowl, combine the flax seed powder with water and allow soaking for 5 minutes.
4. Add the flax egg to the cheese mixture, the crumbled tofu, salt, and black pepper, and combine well. Use your hands to form large meatballs out of the mix.
5. Melt the vegan butter in a large skillet over medium heat and fry the tofu balls until cooked and golden brown on all sides, 10 minutes.
6. Serve the tofu balls with your favorite mashes or in burgers.

Nutrition
- Calories 280
- Fat 3,8g
- Carbs 44.6g
- Protein 0.7g

Greek-style Gigante Beans

Preparation Time: 8 hours 5 minutes
Cooking Time:: 10 hours
Servings: 10

Ingredients:
- 12 ounces gigante beans
- 1 can tomatoes with juice, chopped
- 2 stalks celery, diced
- 1 onion, diced
- 4 garlic cloves, minced
- Salt, to taste

Directions:
1. Soak beans in water for 8 hours.
2. Combine drained beans with the remaining ingredients. Stir, and pour water to cover.
3. Cook for 10 hours on low. Season with salt, and serve.

Nutrition:

- Calories 63
- Carbohydrates 13 g
- Fats 2 g
- Protein 4 g

Brown Rice & Red Beans & Coconut Milk

Preparation Time: 10 minutes
Cooking Time:: 1 hour
Servings: 6

Ingredients:

- 2 cups brown rice, uncooked
- 4 cups water
- 1 Tbsp olive oil
- 1 onion, diced
- 3 cloves garlic, minced
- 2 cans red beans
- 1 can coconut milk

Directions:

1. Bring brown rice in water to a boil, then simmer for 30 minutes.
2. Sauté onion in olive oil. Add garlic and cook until golden.

3.Mix the onions and garlic, beans, and coconut milk into the rice. Simmer for 15 minutes.

4.Serve hot.

Nutrition:
- Calories 280
- Carbohydrates 49 g
- Fats 3 g
- Protein 8 g

Black-Eyed Peas with Herns

Preparation Time: 10 minutes

Cooking Time:: 1 hour

Servings: 8

Ingredients:

- 2 cans no-sodium black-eyed beans
- ½ cup extra-virgin olive oil
- 1 cup parsley, chopped
- 4 green onions, sliced
- 2 carrots, grated
- 2 Tbsp tomato paste
- 2 cups water
- Salt, pepper, to taste

Directions:

1. Drain the beans, reserve the liquid.
2. Sauté beans, parsley, onions, and carrots in oil for 3 minutes.

3. Add remaining ingredients, 2 cups reserved beans liquid, and water.

4. Cook for 30 minutes.

5. Season with salt, pepper and serve.

Nutrition:
- Calories 230
- Carbohydrates 23 g
- Fats 15 g
- Protein 11 g

Cream of Mushroom Soup

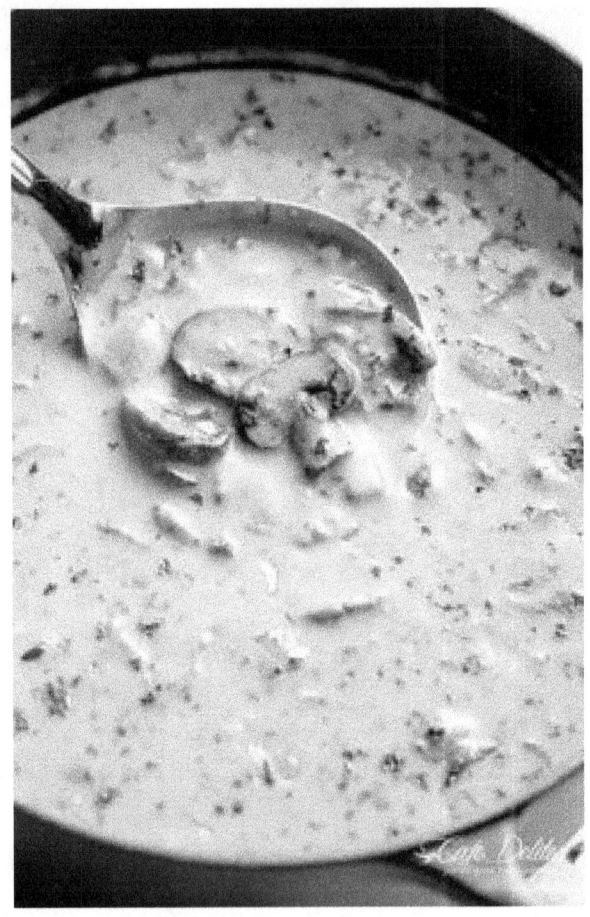

Preparation time: 5 minutes

Cooking time: 12 minutes

Servings: 6

Ingredients:

- 1 medium white onion, peeled, chopped
- 16 ounces button mushrooms, sliced
- 1 ½ teaspoon minced garlic
- 1/4 cup all-purpose flour
- 1/2 teaspoon ground black pepper
- 1 teaspoon dried thyme
- 1/4 teaspoon nutmeg
- 1/2 teaspoon salt
- 2 tablespoons vegan butter
- 4 cups vegetable broth
- 1 1/2 cups coconut milk, unsweetened

Directions:

1. Take a large pot, place it over medium-high heat, add butter and when it melts, add onions and garlic, stir in garlic and cook for 5 minutes until softened and nicely brown.
2. Then sprinkle flour over vegetables, continue cooking for 1 minute, then add remaining ingredients, stir until mixed and simmer for 5 minutes until thickened.
3. Serve straight away

Nutrition:

- Calories: 120 Cal
- Fat: 7 g
- Carbs: 10 g
- Protein: 2 g
- Fiber: 6 g

Cauliflower and Horseradish Soup

Preparation time: 5 minutes
Cooking time: 20 minutes
Servings: 4

Ingredients:

- 2 medium potatoes, peeled, chopped
- 1 medium cauliflower, florets and stalk chopped
- 1 medium white onion, peeled, chopped
- 1 teaspoon minced garlic
- 2/3 teaspoon salt
- 1/3 teaspoon ground black pepper
- 4 teaspoons horseradish sauce
- 1 teaspoon dried thyme
- 3 cups vegetable broth
- 1 cup coconut milk, unsweetened

Directions:

1. Place all the vegetables in a large pan, place it over

medium-high heat, add thyme, pour in broth and milk and bring the mixture to boil.

2.Then switch heat to medium level, simmer the soup for 15 minutes and remove the pan from heat.

3.Puree the soup by using an immersion blender until smooth, season with salt and black pepper, and serve straight away.

Nutrition:
- Calories: 160 Cal
- Fat: 2.6 g
- Carbs: 31 g
- Protein: 6 g
- Fiber: 6 g

Curry Lentil Soup

Preparation time: 5 minutes

Cooking time: 40 minutes

Servings: 6

Ingredients:
1. 1 cup brown lentils
2. 1 medium white onion, peeled, chopped
3. 28 ounces diced tomatoes
4. 1 ½ teaspoon minced garlic
5. 1 inch of ginger, grated
6. 3 cups vegetable broth
7. 1/2 teaspoon salt
8. 2 tablespoons curry powder
9. 1 teaspoon cumin
10. 1/2 teaspoon cayenne
11. 1 tablespoon olive oil
12. 1 1/2 cups coconut milk, unsweetened
13. ¼ cup chopped cilantro
14.

Directions:

1. Take a soup pot, place it over medium-high heat, add oil and when hot, add onion, stir in garlic and ginger and cook for 5 minutes until golden brown.
2. Then add all the ingredients except for milk and cilantro, stir until mixed and simmer for 25 minutes until lentils have cooked.
3. When done, stir in milk, cook for 5 minutes until thoroughly heated and then garnish the soup with cilantro.
4. Serve straight away

Nutrition:

- Calories: 269 Cal
- Fat: 15 g
- Carbs: 26 g
- Protein: 10 g
- Fiber: 10 g

Chickpea Noodle Soup

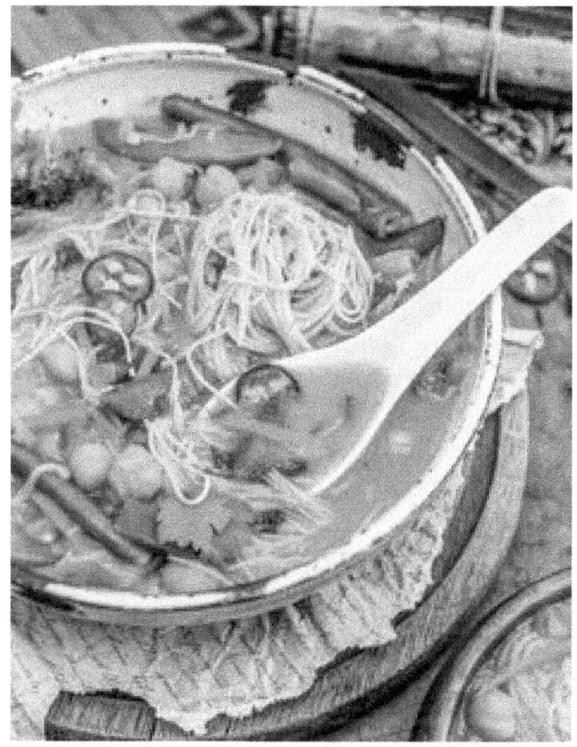

Preparation time: 5 minutes

Cooking time: 18 minutes

Servings: 6

Ingredients:

- 1 cup cooked chickpeas
- 8 ounces rotini noodles, whole-wheat

- 4 celery stalks, sliced
- 2 medium white onions, peeled, chopped
- 4 medium carrots, peeled, sliced
- 2 teaspoons minced garlic
- 8 sprigs of thyme
- 1 teaspoon salt
- 1/3 teaspoon ground black pepper
- 1 bay leaf
- 2 tablespoons olive oil
- 2 quarts of vegetable broth
- ¼ cup chopped fresh parsley

Directions:

1. Take a large pot, place it over medium heat, add oil and when hot, add all the vegetables, stir in garlic, thyme and bay leaf and cook for 5 minutes until vegetables are golden and sauté.
2. Then pour in broth stir and bring the mixture to boil.
3. Add chickpeas and noodles into boiling soup, continue cooking for 8 minutes until noodles are tender, and then season soup with salt and black pepper.

4. Garnish with parsley and serve straight away

Nutrition:

- Calories: 260 Cal
- Fat: 5 g
- Carbs: 44 g
- Protein: 7 g
- Fiber: 4 g

www.ingramcontent.com/pod-product-compliance
Lightning Source LLC
Chambersburg PA
CBHW071110030426
42336CB00013BA/2029